Ultimate

Air Fryer Recipes

Stay Healthy without Worry with Air
Fryer Tasty Recipes for Creative
Meals. Quick and Easy Fried Food!

Ricky Ward

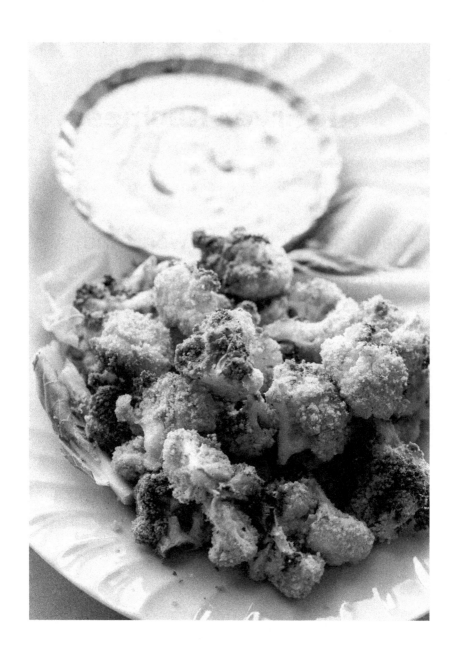

Table of Contents

INTRODUCTION

An air fryer is a kitchen appliance designed to deliver a tasty, crispy, golden-brown morsel of food without the use of oil or other cooking fats. It uses hot air instead of oil or other cooking fats to cook food quickly and evenly.

The air fryer can be used for making fried chips in addition to other foods.

There are several varieties of air fryers. One of the main categories is made up of countertop air fryers designed for individual use in the kitchen. These models sit on the worktop or counter top and feature a basket that sits on a wire rack. This forms the base that holds hot air that cooks food as it passes through it.

air fryer's air fryers are designed to help you make healthy and filling meals. Our electric fryers are perfect for people who want fresh, homemade fries without all of the fat. Our air fryer features a light-weight aluminum design that lets you move the appliance from room to room without worry. Each air fryer is also equipped with a thermostat, making it easy to adjust the temperature as needed.

An air fryer is an appliance that cooks food using high-speed air circulation. It is a perfect alternative to deep frying, baking or roasting, and works great for cooking fast and healthy meals.

How Does an Air Fryer Work?

The fan draws warm air from the bottom of the chamber, which rises and cools as it circulates. The food is then placed in the middle of the basket, and the fan circulates air around it, cooking it all at once. Food cooks faster than if you fried it in oil or baked it in an oven. The food doesn't become soggy like fried food does, either. Because the air circulates around the food rather than through it, you can use much less oil in your Air Fryer. Best of all, since no oil is being used for cooking, there's much less of an environmental impact!

What Types of Air Fryers are Available?

Air fryers come in a variety of sizes as well as different colors and designs. You may find one that has a View Master-like chrome trim or one with a retro design pattern that blends easily into your décor. Some Air fryers are as small as a rice cooker while others can be used to make large batches of French fries with recipes you create on your tablet! Some Air Fryer models have "smart" features that allow you to cook multiple foods at the same time; others have timers so you can automatically set them for particular times during the day. All versions sterilize their own cooking plates by running them through a clean cycle between batches!

When you are looking for a new air fryer, you should take a look at air fryer Cookware. We have all of the features you are looking for in an air fryer, including built in racks that will allow you to cook a full size meal for your family. We also have a variety of accessories that will give you an even better cooking experience.

We are proud to introduce air fryer Cookware, the premier brand in air fryers. You can rest assured that we only use the best materials to ensure our products will work for years to come. Our air fryers feature built-in racks, so you can cook a full-size meal at once. They also include an adjustable thermostat that ranges from 120 to 500 degrees Fahrenheit.

Whether you are looking to impress your family with gourmet French fries or just want to make your favorite chicken drumsticks and vegetables, air fryer Cookware has everything you need. Every item has been carefully tested to ensure safe and responsible use. All of our products carry a One Year Limited Manufacturer Warranty, so you can be confident that they will serve your needs well.

Dehydrated Candied Bacon

Preparation time: 3 hours

Cooking time: 4 hours and 10 minutes

Servings: 4

Ingredients:

- 6 slices bacon
- 3 tablespoons light brown sugar
- 2 tablespoons rice vinegar
- 2 tablespoons chili paste
- 1 tablespoon soy sauce

Directions:

1. Mix brown sugar, rice vinegar, chili paste, and soy sauce together in a bowl.
2. Add bacon slices and mix until all are evenly coated.
3. Set aside for up to 3 hours or up until ready to dehydrate.
4. Then put the bacon on the food tray.
5. Set bacon on the air fryer 's wire rack, then insert the rack at mid-position in the air fryer toaster oven.

6. Select the Dehydrate function on the Air Fryer, set time to 4 hours, then press Start.

7. Remove the tray once done baking and let the bacon cool for 5 minutes, then serve.

Nutrition: Calories 137, Total Fat 8.8g, Total Carbs 6.9g, Protein 7.6g

Dehydrated Spiced Orange Slices

Preparation time: 10 minutes

Cooking time: 6 hours

Servings: 3

Ingredients:

- 2 large oranges, cut into ⅛-inch-thick slices
- ½ teaspoon ground star anise
- ½ teaspoon ground cinnamon
- 1 tbsp Choco-hazelnut spread

Directions:

1. Dash seasonings on the orange slices.
2. Place into the fry basket, then insert the basket at mid-position in the Air Fryer.
3. Select the Dehydrate function, fix the time to 6 hours and temperature to 140°F, then press Start.
4. Remove once done, and if desired serve with chocolate hazelnut spread.

Nutrition: Calories 99, Total Fat 2.2g, Total Carbs 18.2g, Protein 1.6g

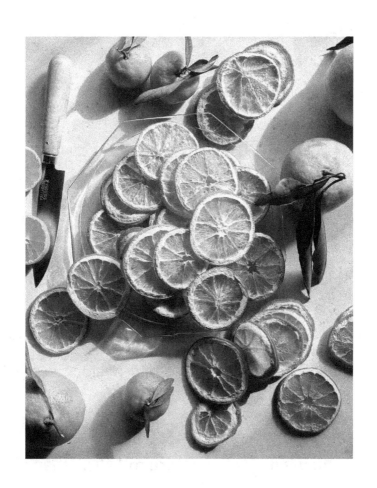

Ranch Kale Chip

Preparation time: 5 minutes

Cooking time: 3 hours

Servings: 2

Ingredients:

- 3 whole kale leaves, cut into 2-inch squares
- 1 tbsp. olive oil
- 1 tbsp. ranch seasoning

Directions:

1. In a small bowl, mix the olive oil and ranch seasoning.
2. Mix ranch mixture with kale leaves until all are evenly coated.
3. Put the kale leaves into the fry basket, then insert the fry basket at mid-position in the Air Fryer.
4. Select the Dehydrate function, fix the time to 3 hours and temperature to 140°F, then press Start/Cancel.
5. Remove when done and serve.

Nutrition: Calories 117, Total Fat 7g, Total Carbs 10.5g, Protein 3g

Taco Seasoned Kale Chips

Preparation time: 5 minutes

Cooking time: 3 hours

Servings: 2

Ingredients:

- 3 whole kale leaves, cut into 2-inch squares
- 1 tbsp.olive oil
- 1 tbsp. taco seasoning

Directions:

1. Mix taco seasoning and olive oil in a small bowl.
2. Combine taco seasoning mixture with kale leaves until all are evenly coated.
3. Place kale leaves into the fry basket, then insert the fry basket at mid-position in the Air Fryer.
4. Select the Dehydrate function, fix the time to 3 hours and temperature to 140°F, then press Start.
5. Remove when done and serve.

Nutrition: Calories 125, Total Fat 7g, Total Carbs 12.5g, Protein 3g

Bacon-Wrapped Hot Dogs

Preparation time: 5 minutes

Cooking time: 20 minutes

Servings: 4

Ingredients:

- 4 strips thick-cut bacon
- 4 beef hot dogs
- 4 hot dog buns, slightly toasted

Directions:

1. Wrap 1 piece of bacon around each hot dog, allowing the edges of the bacon to overlap slightly. Set aside.

2. Select the Broil function on the Air Fryer, fix the time to 20 minutes, then press Start/Cancel to preheat.

3. Line the food tray with foil, then set the wire rack on top of the food tray.

4. Place the bacon-wrapped hot dogs on the wire rack, then insert the rack and food tray at top position in the preheated air fryer toaster oven. Press Start/Cancel.

5. Flip the hot dogs halfway through cooking.

6. Remove when done and place each hot dog in a hot dog bun.

7. Serve with your choice of toppings.

Nutrition: Calories 265, Total Fat 13g, Total Carbs 24g, Protein 13g

Garlic Bread

Preparation time: 5 minutes

Cooking time: 1 hour and 5 minutes

Servings: 2

Ingredients:

- Two 6-inch baguettes halved lengthwise
- 3 tablespoons unsalted butter, melted
- 3 cloves garlic, minced
- ¼ teaspoon salt
- 1 teaspoon dried parsley

Directions:

1. Mix melted butter, minced garlic, salt, and parsley.
2. Brush mixture over each baguette half.
3. Place baguettes on the Air Fryer Toaster Oven's wire rack and insert at mid position.
4. Select the Toast function, set to darkness level 6, and press Start/Cancel.
5. Remove when done and serve immediately

Nutrition: Calories 271, Total Fat 17.7g, Total Carbs 23.5g, Protein 4.5g

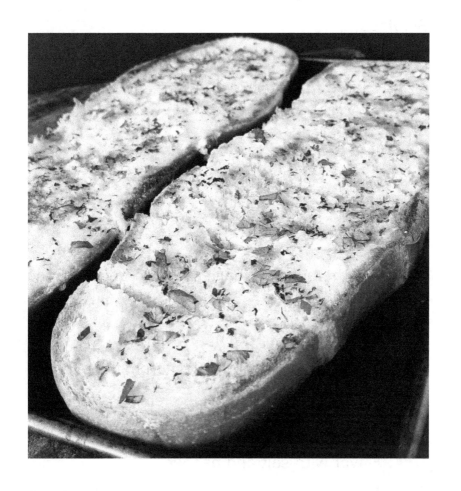

Avocado Baked Egg

Preparation time: 5 minutes

Cooking time: 20 minutes

Servings: 2

Ingredients:

- 1 large ripe avocado, halved and pitted
- 2 eggs
- ¼ tsp. salt
- ¼ tsp. black pepper
- 2 tbsp. grated Parmesan cheese

Directions:

1. Put the avocado halves on the edges of the baking sheet. The rim of the baking sheet will stop them from rolling over.
2. Scoop out some of the flesh from the avocado halves to make a hole large enough for 1 egg.
3. Crack 1 egg into each of the halved avocados.
4. Flavor with salt and pepper.
5. Insert the wire rack at mid-position in the Air Fryer Toaster Oven. Select the Air Fry

function, set timer to 22 minutes, then press Start to warm it up.

6. In the preheated air fryer, place the baking sheet on top of the wire rack then press Start.

7. After 12 minutes of cook time, sprinkle Parmesan cheese on the avocado halves.

8. Remove the baked avocados when done and garnish with finely chopped chives, then serve.

Nutrition: Calories 377, Total Fat 30gTotal Carbs 10.2g, Protein 16.5g

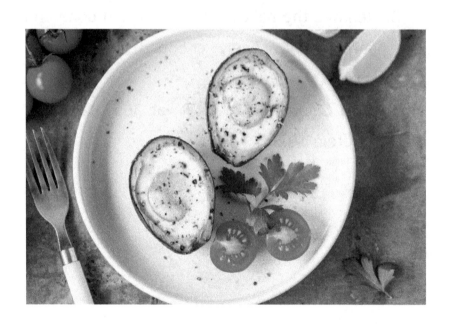

Rotisserie Chicken

Preparation time: 1 hour and 5 minutes

Cooking time: 1 hour and 10 minutes

Servings: 4

Ingredients:

- 1 whole chicken (5 pounds)
- 1-gallon water
- ¾ c.kosher salt
- 3 tbsp.black pepper
- 2 bay leaves

Directions:

1. Mix salt, black pepper, water, and bay leaves to make a brine. Dip the chicken in the mixture and allow to sit for 1 hour.
2. Pat chicken dry, then bind with butcher's twine to ensure the wings and legs are held together.
3. Insert the rotisserie tube through the chicken, securing the chicken between the forks. Put the shaft into the designated ports in the Air Fryer.

4. Choose the Rotisserie function, fix the time to 1 hour 10 minutes and temperature to 380°F, then press Start/. Turn on the high speed for better crispness.

5. Remove rotisserie chicken when done. Carve the chicken into preferred portions, then serve.

Nutrition: Calories 82, Total Fat 2.8g, Total Carbs 3.3g, Protein 10.8g

Air Fryer Buffalo Mushroom Poppers

Preparation Time: 5 minutes

Cooking Time: 10 minutes

Servings: 4

Ingredients:

- 1 pound Sparkling Total Button Mushroom
- ½ cup flour and panko mixture
- Grind Salt and Black Pepper
- 1/4 cup buffalo style hot sauce
- 2 eggs

Directions:

1. Remove the stems from the mushroom peel. Finely chop; Put the cap on one side. Stir the chopped mushroom stem, salt, and pepper together in a small bowl. Fill each mushroom cap with about 1 tablespoon combination, rounding the filling to form a clean ball.

2. Place Pancho in a shallow bowl. Place the dough in a 2d shallow bowl, and the eggs in a third shallow bowl. Coat mushrooms in

flour, dip in egg mixture, and dredge in panko, pressing to adhere. Coat mushrooms properly with cooking spray.

3. Place half of the mushrooms in an air fryer basket, and cook dinner at 350 ° F until golden brown and crispy. Transfer the cooked mushrooms to a huge bowl. Repeat with the last mushroom. Drizzle sauce over mushrooms; toss to coat. Sprinkle with chives.

4. Serve Mushroom Poppers.

Nutrition: Calories: 130 Carbs: 8 g Fat: 6 g Protein: 9 g

Air Fryer Potato Chips

Preparation Time: 5 minutes

Cooking Time: 10 minutes

Servings: 4

Ingredients:

- 1 medium russet potato, peeled,
- 1/8-inch-thick slices (about 3/4 lb.)
- 1 tbsp canola oil
- sea salt and freshly ground black pepper
- 1 tablespoon chopped Happened. Clean henna

Directions:

1. Soak the potato slices in a large bowl of cold water, for 20 minutes. Pat dry the potatoes with paper towels.
2. Dry-wipe the bowl; Then add oil, salt, and pepper. Add potatoes; Toss gently to coat.
3. Lightly grease air fryer basket with cooking spray. Place half a slice of potato in a basket, and prepare dinner in two batches at 375 ° F,

until it becomes crispy within about 25 to 30 minutes.

4. Cautiously remove the chips from the air fryer to the plate using a pair of tongs, Sprinkle over rosemary; Shop once or in an airtight plastic container.

Nutrition: Calories: 110 Carbs: 7 g Fat: 6 g Protein: 7 g

Air Fried Corn Dog Bites

Preparation Time: 5 minutes

Cooking Time: 10 minutes

Servings: 4

Ingredients:

- 2 uncured All Beef Hot Puppies
- ½ cup All-Purpose Flour
- Half Cup Bamboo Broach (About 2 1/8 oz.) or 12 craft sticks
- 1 1/2 cups minced corn flakes cereal
- 2 large eggs, lightly beaten

Directions:

1. Slice each hot dog half lengthwise each length. Cut each half into 3 equal pieces. Put a craft stick or bamboo skewer at 1 end of each piece of a hot dog.

2. Place the dough in a shallow dish. Place the overwhelmed eggs gently in another shallow dish. Place the cornflakes in a 0.33 shallow dish. Dip the hot dogs in the flour, adding extra. Dip in eggs, allowing any excess to drip

off. Dredge into cornflake pieces, pressing to adhere.

3. Lightly grease the air fryer basket with cooking spray. Place 6 corn dog bites in a basket; Spray lightly with cooking spray. Cook at 375 ° F until the corn is golden brown and crispy, 10 minutes, cut the corn dog through cooking. Repeat with remaining corn dog bite.

4. To serve, place three corn dog bites on each plate with 2 tablespoons of mustard, and serve immediately.

Nutrition: Calories: 190 Carbs: 10 g Fat: 8 g Protein: 15 g

Sauté in an Air Fryer

Preparation Time: 5 minutes

Cooking Time: 20 minutes

Servings: 4

Ingredients:

- Empanadas 1 tablespoon olive oil 3 ounces (85/15) lean floor red meat 1/4 cup finely chopped white onion three ounces.
- Finely cremini mushrooms 2 tablespoons chopped finely garlic 6 pitted green olives chopped, cinnamon half cup chopped tomatoes chopped
- 1/4 red bell pepper
- 1/4 teaspoon ground cumin
- 1/8 teaspoon ground 8 square gyoza wrappers 1 large egg, beaten gently

Directions:

1. In a medium pan, heat the oil on medium-high. Add beef and onion; Baking, crumble, until beginning to brown, three minutes.

2. Add mushrooms; Cook, stirring occasionally until the mushrooms are beginning to brown, 6 minutes. Add garlic, olives, paprika, cumin, and cinnamon; Cook the dinner until the mushrooms become very soft and leave their liquid for 3 minutes. Stir in tomatoes, and cook dinner 1 minute, stirring occasionally. Transfer the filling to a bowl, and let cool for 5 minutes.

3. Arrange the 4 goji covers on the work surface. Place about 1 tbsp of stuffing in the center of each cover. Brush the edges of the wrapper with eggs; Wrap the folds, wrapping the edges to seal. Repeat technique with closing cover and filling.

4. Place 4 implants in one layer in an air fryer basket, and cook for 7 minutes, until well browned at 400 ° F. Repeat with the last empanadas.

Nutrition: Calories: 220 Carbs: 12 g Fat: 10 g Protein: 19 g

Air Fryer Churros with Chocolate Sauce

Preparation Time: 5 minutes

Cooking Time: 10 minutes

Servings: 4

Ingredients:

- 1/2 cup water 1/4 teaspoon kosher salt
- Unsalted butter, split half cup
- 2 tbsp. All-purpose flour
- 2 large eggs
- 1/3 cup granulated sugar cinnamon

Directions:

1. Bring 1/4 cup of water, salt, and butter to a boil in a small saucepan over medium-high. Reduce heat from medium to low; Add the flour, and stir vigorously with a wooden spoon until the dough is smooth about 30 seconds.

2. Continue cooking, stirring continuously, until the dough starts to move away from the sides of the pan and leave a movie variety on the back of the pan for 2 to 3 minutes.

3. Transfer the dough to a medium bowl. Stir continuously for about 1 minute, until slightly cooled. Add eggs, 1 at a time, stirring continuously until completely smooth after each addition. Transfer the mixture to a piping bag equipped with a medium celebrity tip. Chill 30 minutes.

4. Pipe 6 (3 inches long) pieces into one layer in an air fryer basket. Cook at 380 ° F, about 10 minutes, until golden. Repeat with the last flour.

5. In a medium bowl, collectively stir the sugar and cinnamon. Brush the cooked churros with the remaining 2 tablespoons of melted butter, and roll in a sugar mixture.

6. Serve churros with chocolate sauce.

Nutrition: Calories: 108 Fat:6 Carbs: 12 Protein:1

Air Fryer Sweet Potato Tots

Preparation Time: 5 minutes

Cooking Time: 10 minutes

Servings: 4

Ingredients:

- 2 small (14 ounces total) candy potatoes, peeled
- 1 tbsp potato starch
- 1/8 teaspoon garlic powder
- 1 1/4 teaspoons kosher salt, split 3/4 cup no salt

Directions:

1. Put a medium pan of water to a boil over high heat. Add the potatoes, and cook the dinner until the fork is tender about 15 minutes. Transfer potatoes to a plate to cool for about 15 minutes.

2. Working on a medium bowl, grate a potato using a giant hole in a box grater. Gently toss with potato starch, garlic powder, and 1 teaspoon salt. Size combination in

approximately 24 (1-inch) total-shaped cylinders.

3. Lightly grease the air fryer with cooking spray. Put 1/2 of the children (about 12) in a layer in the basket, and spray with cooking spray. Cook to 400 ° F for 12 to 14 minutes, turning the children halfway through the Cooking Time. Remove from the fry basket and sprinkle with 1/8 teaspoon salt. Repeat with remaining children and salt. Serve directly with ketchup.

Nutrition: Calories: 120 Carbs: 7 g Fat: 5 g Protein: 8 g

Air-Fried Calzone

Preparation Time: 5 minutes

Cooking Time: 20 minutes

Servings: 4

Ingredients:

- 1 teaspoon olive oil
- 1/4 cup finely chopped pink onion (from 1 small onion) 3 oz.
- Baby spinach leaves (about three cups) 1/3 cup low-sodium marinara sauce 2 oz.
- Chopped rotisserie hen breast (about 1/3 cup)
- 1 1/2 ounces' flour 6 ounces freshly prepared wheat pizza pre-chopped (about 6 Karachi.) Part-time skim mozzarella cheese spray cooking

Directions:

1. heat the olive oil in a medium nonstick pan on medium-high. Add onion, stirring occasionally, until tender, and cook for 2 minutes. Add spinach; Cook for two and a half

minutes, until dinner is covered. Remove pan from heat; Stir in marinara sauce and chicken.

2. Divide flour into 4 equal pieces. Gently roll each piece into a 6-inch circle on a flared surface. Place one-quarter of the spinach mixture more than half of each flour cycle. Top with one-quarter cheese. To bend the dough, fold the dough, shrink the seal. Coat calzone with cooking spray.

3. Place the calzone in an air fryer basket, and prepare dinner at 325 ° F for 12 minutes, until the dough turns golden brown, flip the calzone after eight minutes.

Nutrition: Calories: 260 Carbs: 17 g Fat: 13 g Protein: 24 g

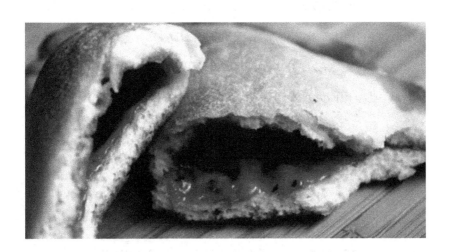

Air-Fried Buffalo Cauliflower Bites

Preparation Time: 5 minutes

Cooking Time: 30 minutes

Servings: 4

Ingredients:

- 3 tablespoons ketchup without salt 2 tablespoons hot sauce (e.g. Frank's Red-hot)
- 1 giant egg white 3/4 cup Panko (Japanese-style cream) 1/2 (3-lb) Head.
- Cauliflower, trimmed and cooked in 1-inch florets (about 4 cups of florets).
- Cooking spray 1/4 cup low-fat buttercream 1/4-ounce crumbled blue cheese (about 1 tbsp) 1 small garlic clove, 1 teaspoon pink wine. Vinegar 1/4 teaspoon pepper.

Directions:

1. In a small bowl, collectively ketchup, hot sauce, and egg whites until smooth. Place panko in a large bowl. Toss the cauliflower flower and ketchup combination collectively into another giant bowl until coated. Working

in batches, tossing cauliflower to coat the panko. Coat cabbage well with cooking spray.

2. Put the cabbage in an air fryer basket, and cook at 320 ° F for about 20 minutes, until golden brown and crisp. Repeat with the remaining cauliflower.

3. When the cabbage cooks, stir together bitter cream, blue cheese, garlic, vinegar and pepper in a small bowl. Serve the cabbage with blue cheese sauce.

Nutrition: Calories: 140 Carbs: 9 g Fat: 6 g Protein: 10 g

Artichoke Chicken

Preparation time: 15 minutes

Cooking time: 50 minutes

Servings: 8

Ingredients:

- 8 boneless skinless chicken breast halves
- 2 tbsp. of butter
- 2 jars (6 oz. each) marinated quartered artichoke hearts, drained
- 1 jar (4½ oz.) whole mushrooms, drained
- ½ cup of chopped onion
- 1/3 cup all-purpose flour
- 1½ tsp. of dried rosemary, crushed
- ¾ tsp. of salt
- ¼ tsp. of pepper
- 2 cups of chicken broth or (1 cup of broth and 1 cup of dry white wine)
- Hot cooked noodles
- Fresh parsley, minced

Directions:

1. In a large skillet, brown the chicken in butter. After browning chicken, remove chicken to an ungreased 13x9-in. baking dish.
2. Then arrange artichokes and mushrooms on top of chicken and set aside. Sauté the onion in pan juices (until crisp-tender).
3. In a bowl, mix the rosemary, flour, salt and pepper. Stir into pan until blended.
4. Add in the chicken broth and bring to a boil, cook and stir constantly until thickened and bubbly, for about 1 to 2 minutes.
5. Remove from the heat, spoon over chicken and uncovered at 350° until a thermometer inserted in the chicken reads 170°, for about 35 to 40 minutes.
6. Serve with pasta and sprinkle with parsley. Serve and enjoy!

Nutrition: Calories: 280 Carbs: 19 g Fat: 15 g Protein: 28 g

Quentin's Peach-Bourbon Wings

Preparation Time: 35 minutes

Cooking Time: 15 minutes

Serving: 2

Ingredients:

- ½ cup of peach preserves
- 1 tbsp. of brown sugar
- 1 garlic clove, minced
- ¼ tsp. of salt
- 2 tbsp. of white vinegar
- 2 tbsp. of bourbon
- 1 tsp. of corn starch
- 1½ tsp. of water
- 2 lb. of chicken wings

Directions:

1. Start by heating your Air fryer to 400°F. Place the preserves, brown sugar, garlic and salt in a food processor, process until blended.
2. After blending the mixture, transfer to a small saucepan. Add vinegar and bourbon, bring to a boil.

3. Reduce heat, simmer, uncovered, until slightly thickened, for about 4 to 6 minutes.

4. Mix water and cornstarch in a bowl, until smooth. Stir into preserve mixture.

5. Return to a boil. Cook and stir constantly for about 1 to 2 minutes (until thickened).

6. Reserve ¼ cup of sauce for serving. Use a sharp knife, cut through the two joints on each chicken wing.

7. Discard wing tips. Grease the basket of your Air fryer with cooking oil. (Work in batches as needed).

8. Place chicken wing pieces in a single layer in the basket of your Air fryer. Set your Air fryer to cook for about 6 minutes.

9. After the 6 minutes, turn and brush with preserve mixture. Return to your Air fryer, cook until browned and juices run clear, for about 6 to 8 minutes longer.

10.   Remove and keep warm. Repeat with remaining wing pieces.

11.   Serve wings immediately with reserved
    sauce.

12.   Serve and enjoy!

Nutrition: Calories: 170 Carbs: 11 g Fat: 9 g
Protein: 17 g

Chicken Breast

Preparation time: 5 minutes

Cooking time: 15 minutes

Servings: 4

Ingredients:

- 5 to 6 oz. chicken breasts split in half lengthwise
- Seasoning salt of choice
- Salt and pepper to taste

Directions:

1. Set the Air fryer to 400°F. Cut the chicken breast in half and flavor with salt and pepper.
2. Place the chicken in the basket of your Air fryer, set the temperature to 400°F.
3. Close the basket and set the timer to cook for about 7 minutes. When the time is up.
4. Take the chicken out and flip, cook for another 4 minutes longer.
5. After the 4 minutes, remove and serve.
6. Serve immediately and enjoy.

Nutrition: Calories: 250 Carbs: 16 g Fat: 12 g
Protein: 25 g

Rotisserie Style Whole Chicken

Preparation time: 5 minutes

Cooking time: 1 hour

Servings: 4

Ingredients:

- 1 whole chicken cleaned and blotted dry
- 2 tbsp. of Ghee (or coconut or olive oil)
- 1 tbsp. of TOG house seasoning

Directions:

1. Remove giblet packet from chicken and pat dry. Rub Ghee/Oil all over the chicken. Season generously with TOG house seasoning.
2. Place the chicken breast side down into your Air fryer. Set timer to cook at 350°F for about 30 minutes.
3. After the 30 minutes, flip chicken over and cook at 350°F for an additional 30 minutes.
4. Once the cooking is done, let rest for about 10 minutes.
5. Serve immediately and enjoy!

Nutrition: Calories: 350 Carbs: 24 g Fat: 21 g Protein: 42 g

Greek Stuffed Chicken Breast

Preparation time: 10 minutes

Cooking time: 15 minutes

Servings: 4

Ingredients:

- 26-oz. boneless skinless chicken breasts
- 1 cup of wild rice, prepared
- 4 oz. fat-free feta cheese
- 4 tbsp. of `Greek salad dressing

Directions:

1. Slice the chicken breasts in half, making a total of 4 pieces of chicken.
2. Between two pieces of parchment paper, pound the chicken breasts until thin.
3. Mix prepared wild rice, 1 tbsp. of Greek dressing, and fat-free feta cheese together in a medium mixing bowl.
4. Place ¼ rice mixture onto center of each chicken breast and roll covering mixture.
5. Place each chicken breasts rolled side down into your Air fryer pan. Brush the remaining

Greek dressing over the tops of your chicken breasts.

6. Set timer to cook at 382°F for about 15 minutes. When the time is up.

7. Serve immediately and enjoy!

Nutrition: Calories: 280 Carbs: 18 g Fat: 13 g Protein: 27 g

Air Fried Buffalo Chicken Strips

Preparation time: 5 minutes

Cooking time: 15 minutes

Servings: 4

Ingredients:

- 12 ounces chicken breast strips
- ¼ cup of flour
- 1 egg (or liquid egg whites)
- Buffalo Sauce - (We used about 1/2 cup)
- Garlic salt and pepper to taste

Directions:

1. In a separate bowl, place egg, and flour
2. Spray a little cooking spray on the bottom of your Air fryer. Dip chicken in the flour, and then the egg, until well coated.
3. Place the chicken in your Air fryer, spray the top of the chicken with a little more cooking spray.
4. Set the timer to fry at 375°F for about 10 minutes. After the 10 minutes, flip and cook for an additional 3 to 5 minutes.

5. When the time is up, remove chicken from your Air fryer. Place in a mixing bowl and toss in buffalo sauce until well coated.

6. Serve with celery, carrots and ranch.

7. Serve and enjoy!

Nutrition: Calories: 220 Carbs: 14 g Fat: 10 g Protein: 21 g

Whole30 Lemon Pepper Chicken

Preparation time: 5 minutes

Cooking time: 15 minutes

Servings: 3

Ingredients:

- 1 chicken breast
- 2 lemons rind and juice
- 1 tablespoon of chicken seasoning
- 1 teaspoon of garlic puree
- Salt & pepper

Directions:

1. Start by heating your Air fryer to 180°C. Set up your work station. Place a large sheet of silver foil on the work top.

2. Add all the seasonings to it and the lemon rind. Lay out the chicken breasts onto a chopping board.

3. Trim off any fatty bits and any little bones. Season each side with salt and pepper.

4. Rub the chicken seasoning into both sides of the chicken breast so that it is slightly a different color.

5. Place it in the silver foil sheet, rub it thoroughly so that it is fully seasoned. Seal it up very tight so that it can't breathe.

6. Give it a slap with a rolling pin so that it will flatten it out and release more flavor.

7. Place it in your Air fryer. Set your Air fryer to cook for about 15 minutes. After the 15 minutes, check to see if it is fully cooked in the middle before serving.

8. Serve immediately and enjoy!

Nutrition: Calories: 260 Carbs: 16 g Fat: 13 g Protein: 26 g

Roasted Chicken

Preparation time: 5 minutes

Cooking time: 1 hour and 10 minutes

Servings: 4

Ingredients:

- 1 whole chicken
- 1 tablespoon of avocado oil
- 2 tbsp. of primal palate super gyro seasoning
- 2 tablespoons of primal palate new bae seasoning
- 1 tablespoon of Himalayan pink salt

Directions:

1. Start by heating your Air fryer to 375°F. wash the chicken with clean water and Pat the chicken dry.
2. Drizzle with avocado oil. Season with half the seasonings. Place the whole chicken in the basket of your Air fryer.
3. Set timer to cook for about 30 minutes. Flip the chicken after 30 minutes and add the remaining seasoning.

4. After flipping the chicken, set timer to cook the chicken for another 30 minutes.

5. Once the chicken is done cooking, remove the chicken from the basket.

6. Allow it to cool for about 5 minutes before slicing and serving.

7. Serve and enjoy!

Nutrition: Calories: 330 Carbs: 23 g Fat: 19 g Protein: 39 g

Pizza Stuffed Chicken

Preparation time: 10 minutes

Cooking time: 15 minutes

Servings: 4

Ingredients:

- 5 boneless skinless, chicken thighs
- ½ cup of pizza sauce
- 14 slices of turkey pepperoni
- ½ small red onion sliced
- 5 ounce of sliced mozzarella cheese

Directions:

1. Open the chicken thighs and lay them flat on a piece of parchment paper.
2. Place another piece of parchment paper on top of the chicken. Pound the chicken to create a thin piece.
3. Spoon on a tbsp. of pizza sauce on each piece of the chicken and spread it equally. Put 3 pieces of turkey pepperoni on top of the sauce.

4. Add a slice of Mozzarella cheese. Fold one side of the chicken over on to the other. Use a toothpick to hold the chicken together.

5. Once cooked it stays together on its own. Preheat your Air fryer to 370°F for about 2 minutes.

6. Smear the tray with oil, and lay the pieces out in a single layer. Add the chicken and set you Air fryer to cook for about 6 minutes.

7. After the 6 minutes, Flip the chicken and cook for another 6 minutes. Add the cheese to melt on the top for the last 3 minutes,

8. Always check chicken thighs to ensure they are heated to 165F.

9. When the time is up, serve and enjoy!

Nutrition: Calories: 290 Carbs: 18 g Fat: 15 g Protein: 31 g

Desserts

Perfect Cinnamon Toast

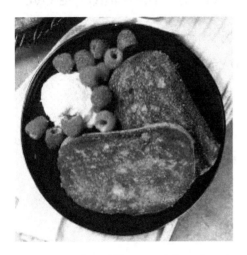

Preparation Time: 10 minutes

Cooking Time: 5 minutes

Servings: 6

Ingredients:

- 2 tsp. pepper
- 1 ½ tsp. cinnamon
- ½ C. sweetener of choice
- 1 C. coconut oil
- 12 slices whole wheat bread

Directions:

1. Melt coconut oil and mix with sweetener until dissolved. Mix in remaining ingredients minus bread till incorporated.
2. Spread mixture onto bread, covering all area.
3. Pour the coated pieces of bread into the Oven rack/basket. Place the Rack on the middle-shelf of the Air fryer oven. Set temperature to 400°F, and set time to 5 minutes.
4. Remove and cut diagonally. Enjoy!

Nutrition: Calories – 124 Protein – 0 g. Fat – 2 g. Carbs – 5 g.

Angel Food Cake

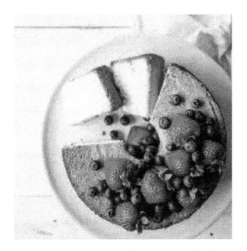

Preparation Time: 5 minutes

Cooking Time: 30 minutes

Servings: 12

Ingredients:

- ¼ cup butter, melted
- 1 cup powdered erythritol
- 1 teaspoon strawberry extract
- 12 egg whites
- 2 teaspoons cream of tartar

Directions:

1. Preheat the air fryer oven for 5 minutes.
2. Blend the cream of tartar and egg whites.

3. Use a hand mixer and whisk until white and fluffy.

4. Add the rest of the ingredients except for the butter and whisk for another minute.

5. Pour into a baking dish.

6. Place in the air fryer basket and cook for 30 minutes at 400°F or if a toothpick inserted in the middle comes out clean.

7. Drizzle with melted butter once cooled.

Nutrition: Calories – 65 Protein – 3.1 g. Fat – 5 g. Carbs – 6.2 g.

Apple Dumplings

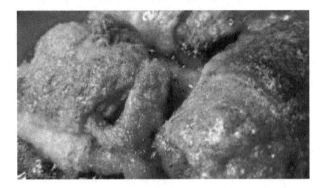

Preparation Time: 10 minutes

Cooking Time: 25 minutes

Servings: 4

Ingredients:

- 2 tbsp. melted coconut oil
- 2 puff pastry sheets
- 1 tbsp. brown sugar
- 2 tbsp. raisins
- 2 small apples of choice

Directions:

1. Ensure your air fryer oven is preheated to 356 degrees.

2. Core and peel apples and mix with raisins and sugar.

3. Place a bit of apple mixture into puff pastry sheets and brush sides with melted coconut oil.

4. Place into the air fryer. Cook 25 minutes, turning halfway through. Will be golden when done.

Nutrition: Calories – 367 Protein – 2 g. Fat – 7 g. Carbs – 10 g.

Chocolate Donuts

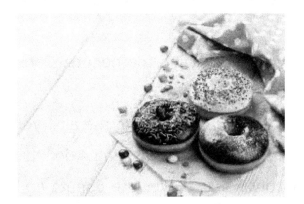

Preparation Time: 5 minutes

Cooking Time: 20 minutes

Servings: 8-10

Ingredients:

- (8-ounce) can jumbo biscuits
- Cooking oil
- Chocolate sauce, such as Hershey's

Directions:

1. Separate the biscuit dough into 8 biscuits and place them on a flat work surface. Use a small circle cookie cutter or a biscuit cutter to cut a hole in the center of each biscuit. You can also cut the holes using a knife.
2. Grease the basket with cooking oil.

3. Place 4 donuts in the air fryer oven. Do not stack. Spray with cooking oil. Cook for 4 minutes.

4. Open the air fryer and flip the donuts. Cook for an additional 4 minutes.

5. Remove the cooked donuts from the air fryer oven, then repeat for the remaining 4 donuts.

6. Drizzle chocolate sauce over the donuts and enjoy while warm.

Nutrition: Calories – 181 Protein – 3 g. Fat – 98 g. Carbs – 42 g.

Apple Hand Pies

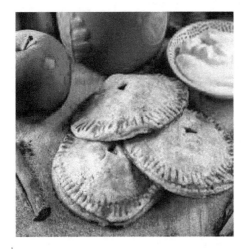

Preparation Time: 5 minutes

Cooking Time: 8 minutes

Servings: 6

Ingredients:

- 15-ounces no-sugar-added apple pie filling
- 1 store-bought crust

Directions:

1. Lay out pie crust and slice into equal-sized squares.

2. Place 2 tbsp. filling into each square and seal crust with a fork.

3. Pour into the Oven rack/basket. Place the Rack on the middle-shelf of the Air fryer oven.

Set temperature to 390°F, and set time to 8 minutes until golden in color.

Nutrition: Calories – 278 Protein – 5 g. Fat – 10 g. Carbs – 17 g.

Sweet Cream Cheese Wontons

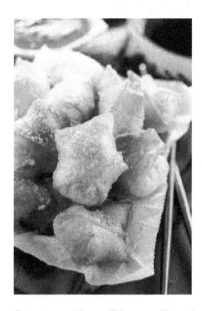

Preparation Time: 5 minutes

Cooking Time: 5 minutes

Servings: 16

Ingredients:

- 1 egg with a little water
- Wonton wrappers
- ½ C. powdered erythritol
- 8 ounces softened cream cheese
- Olive oil

Directions:

1. Mix sweetener and cream cheese together.

2. Lay out 4 wontons at a time and cover with a dish towel to prevent drying out.
3. Place ½ of a teaspoon of cream cheese mixture into each wrapper.
4. Dip finger into egg/water mixture and fold diagonally to form a triangle. Seal edges well.
5. Repeat with remaining ingredients.
6. Place filled wontons into the air fryer oven and cook 5 minutes at 400 degrees, shaking halfway through cooking.

Nutrition: Calories – 303 Protein – 0.5 g. Fat – 3 g. Carbs – 3 g.

French Toast Bites

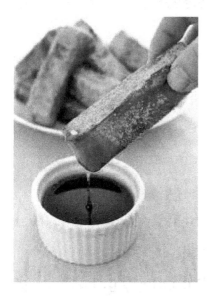

Preparation Time: 5 minutes

Cooking Time: 15 minutes

Servings: 8

Ingredients:

- Almond milk
- Cinnamon
- Sweetener
- 3 eggs
- 4 pieces wheat bread

Directions:

1. Preheat the air fryer oven to 360 degrees.

2. Whisk eggs and thin out with almond milk.

3. Mix 1/3 cup of sweetener with lots of cinnamon.

4. Tear bread in half, ball up pieces and press together to form a ball.

5. Soak bread balls in egg and then roll into cinnamon sugar, making sure to thoroughly coat.

6. Place coated bread balls into the air fryer oven and bake 15 minutes.

Nutrition: Calories – 289 Protein – 0 g. Fat – 11 g. Carbs – 17 g.

Cinnamon Sugar Roasted Chickpeas

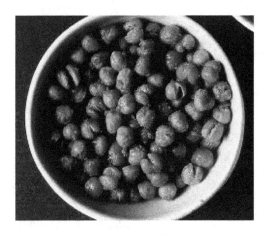

Preparation Time: 5 minutes

Cooking Time: 10 minutes

Servings: 2

Ingredients:

- 1 tbsp. sweetener
- 1 tbsp. cinnamon
- 1 C. chickpeas

Directions:

1. Preheat air fryer oven to 390 degrees.
2. Rinse and drain chickpeas.
3. Mix all ingredients together and add to air fryer.

4. Pour into the Oven rack/basket. Place the Rack on the middle-shelf of the Air fryer oven. Set temperature to 390°F, and set time to 10 minutes.

Nutrition: Calories – 111 Protein – 16 g. Fat – 19 g. Carbs – 18 g.

Brownie Muffins

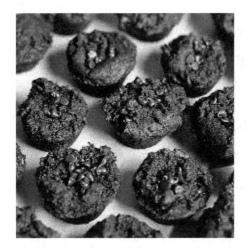

Preparation Time: 10 minutes

Cooking Time: 10 minutes

Servings: 12

Ingredients:

- 1 package Betty Crocker fudge brownie mix
- ¼ cup walnuts, chopped
- 1 egg
- 1/3 cup vegetable oil
- 2 teaspoons water

Directions:

1. Grease 12 muffin molds. Set aside.

2. In a bowl, put all ingredients together.

3. Place the mixture into the prepared muffin molds.

4. Press "Power Button" of Air Fry Oven and turn the dial to select the "Air Fry" mode.

5. Press the Time button and again turn the dial to set the cooking time to 10 minutes.

6. Now push the Temp button and rotate the dial to set the temperature at 300 degrees F.

7. Press "Start/Pause" button to start.

8. When the unit beeps to show that it is preheated, open the lid.

9. Arrange the muffin molds in "Air Fry Basket" and insert in the oven.

10. Place the muffin molds onto a wire rack to cool for about 10 minutes.

11. Carefully, invert the muffins onto the wire rack to completely cool before serving.

Nutrition: Calories – 168 Protein – 2 g. Fat – 8.9 g. Carbs – 20.8 g.

Chocolate Mug Cake

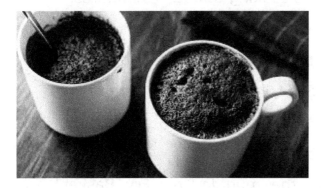

Preparation Time: 15 minutes

Cooking Time: 13 minutes

Servings: 1

Ingredients:

- ¼ cup self-rising flour
- 5 tablespoons caster sugar
- 1 tablespoon cocoa powder
- 3 tablespoons coconut oil
- 3 tablespoons whole milk

Directions:

1. In a shallow mug, add all the ingredients and mix until well combined.
2. Press "Power Button" of Air Fry Oven and turn the dial to select the "Air Fry" mode.

3. Press the Time button and again turn the dial to set the cooking time to 13 minutes.

4. Now push the Temp button and rotate the dial to set the temperature at 392 degrees F.

5. Press "Start/Pause" button to start.

6. When the unit beeps to show that it is preheated, open the lid.

7. Arrange the mug in "Air Fry Basket" and insert in the oven.

8. Place the mug onto a wire rack to cool slightly before serving.

Nutrition: Calories – 729 Protein – 5.7 g. Fat – 43.3 g. Carbs – 88.8 g.

Grilled Peaches

Preparation Time: 10 minutes

Cooking Time: 10 minutes

Servings: 2

Ingredients:

- 2 peaches, cut into wedges and remove pits
- ¼ cup butter, diced into pieces
- ¼ cup brown sugar
- ¼ cup graham cracker crumbs

Directions:

1. Arrange peach wedges on air fryer oven rack and air fry at 350 F for 5 minutes.
2. In a bowl, put the butter, graham cracker crumbs, and brown sugar together.
3. Turn peaches skin side down.
4. Spoon butter mixture over top of peaches and air fry for 5 minutes more.
5. Top with whipped cream and serve.

Nutrition: Calories – 378 Protein – 2.3 g. Fat – 24.4 g. Carbs – 40.5 g.

Simple & Delicious Spiced Apples

Preparation Time: 10 minutes

Cooking Time: 10 minutes

Servings: 4

Ingredients:

- 4 apples, sliced
- 1 tsp apple pie spice
- 2 tbsp sugar
- 2 tbsp ghee, melted

Directions:

1. Add apple slices into the mixing bowl.
2. Add remaining ingredients on top of apple slices and toss until well coated.
3. Transfer apple slices on instant vortex air fryer oven pan and air fry at 350 F for 10 minutes.
4. Top with ice cream and serve.

Nutrition: Calories – 196 Protein – 0.6 g. Fat – 6.8 g. Carbs – 37.1 g.

Tangy Mango Slices

Preparation Time: 10 minutes

Cooking Time: 12 hours

Servings: 6

Ingredients:

- 4 mangoes, peel and cut into ¼-inch slices
- 1/4 cup fresh lemon juice
- 1 tbsp honey

Directions:

1. In a big bowl, combine together honey and lemon juice and set aside.
2. Add mango slices in lemon-honey mixture and coat well.
3. Arrange mango slices on instant vortex air fryer rack and dehydrate at 135 F for 12 hours.

Nutrition: Calories – 147 Protein – 1.9 g. Fat – 0.9 g. Carbs – 36.7 g.

Dried Raspberries

Preparation Time: 10 minutes

Cooking Time: 15 hours

Servings: 4

Ingredients:

- 4 cups raspberries, wash and dry
- 1/4 cup fresh lemon juice

Directions:

1. Add raspberries and lemon juice in a bowl and toss well.

2. Arrange raspberries on instant vortex air fryer oven tray and dehydrate at 135 F for 12-15 hours.

3. Store in an air-tight container.

Nutrition: Calories – 68 Protein – 1.6 g. Fat – 0.9 g. Carbs – 15 g.

Sweet Peach Wedges

Preparation Time: 10 minutes

Cooking Time: 8 hours

Servings: 4

Ingredients:

- 3 peaches, cut and remove pits and sliced
- 1/2 cup fresh lemon juice

Directions:

1. Add lemon juice and peach slices into the bowl and toss well.
2. Arrange peach slices on instant vortex air fryer oven rack and dehydrate at 135 F for 6-8 hours.
3. Serve and enjoy.

Nutrition: Calories – 52 Protein – 1.3 g. Fat – 0.5 g. Carbs – 11.1 g.

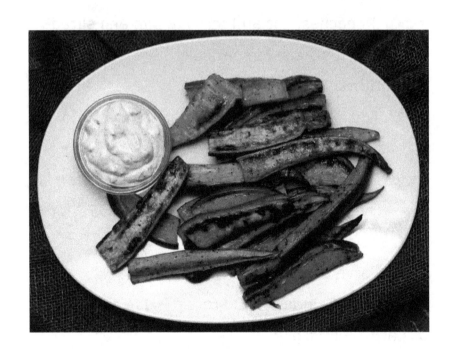

Air Fryer Oreo Cookies

Preparation Time: 5 minutes

Cooking Time: 5 minutes

Servings: 9

Ingredients:

- Pancake Mix: ½ cup
- Water: ½ cup
- Cooking spray
- Chocolate sandwich cookies: 9 (e.g. Oreo)
- Confectioners' sugar: 1 tablespoon, or to taste

Directions:

1. Blend the pancake mixture with the water until well mixed.

2. Line the parchment paper on the basket of an air fryer. Spray nonstick cooking spray on parchment paper. Dip each cookie into the mixture of the pancake and place it in the basket. Make sure they do not touch; if possible, cook in batches.

3. The air fryer is preheated to 400 degrees F (200 degrees C). Add basket and cook for 4 to 5 minutes; flip until golden brown, 2 to 3 more minutes. Sprinkle the sugar over the cookies and serve.

Nutrition: Calories – 77 Protein – 1.2 g. Fat – 2.1 g. Carbs – 13.7 g.

Air Fried Butter Cake

Preparation Time: 10 minutes

Cooking Time: 15 minutes

Servings: 4

Ingredients:

- 7 Tablespoons of butter, at ambient temperature
- White sugar: ¼ cup plus 2 tablespoons
- All-purpose flour: 1 ⅔ cups
- Salt: 1 pinch or to taste
- Milk: 6 tablespoons

Directions:

1. Preheat an air fryer to 350 F (180 C). Spray the cooking spray on a tiny fluted tube pan.
2. Take a large bowl and add ¼ cup butter and 2 tablespoons of sugar in it.
3. Take an electric mixer to beat the sugar and butter until smooth and fluffy. Stir in salt and flour. Stir in the milk and thoroughly combine batter. Move batter to the prepared

saucepan; use a spoon back to level the surface.

4. Place the pan inside the basket of the air fryer. Set the timer within 15 minutes. Bake the batter until a toothpick comes out clean when inserted into the cake.

5. Turn the cake out of the saucepan and allow it to cool for about five minutes.

Nutrition: Calories – 470 Protein – 7.9 g. Fat – 22.4 g. Carbs – 59.7 g.

Air Fryer S'mores

Preparation Time: 5 minutes

Cooking Time: 3 minutes

Servings: 4

Ingredients:

- Four graham crackers (each half split to make 2 squares, for a total of 8 squares)
- 8 Squares of Hershey's chocolate bar, broken into squares
- 4 Marshmallows

Directions:

1. Take deliberate steps. Air-fryers use hot air for cooking food. Marshmallows are light and fluffy, and this should keep the marshmallows from flying around the basket if you follow these steps.
2. Put 4 squares of graham crackers on a basket of the air fryer.
3. Place 2 squares of chocolate bars on each cracker.

4. Place back the basket in the air fryer and fry on air at 390 °F for 1 minute. It is barely long enough for the chocolate to melt. Remove basket from air fryer.

5. Top with a marshmallow over each cracker. Throw the marshmallow down a little bit into the melted chocolate. This will help to make the marshmallow stay over the chocolate.

6. Put back the basket in the air fryer and fry at 390 °F for 2 minutes. (The marshmallows should be puffed up and browned at the tops.)

7. Using tongs to carefully remove each cracker from the basket of the air fryer and place it on a platter. Top each marshmallow with another square of graham crackers.

8. Enjoy it right away!

Nutrition: Calories – 200 Protein – 2.6 g. Fat – 3.1 g. Carbs – 15.7 g.

Peanut Butter Cookies

Preparation Time: 2 minutes

Cooking Time: 5 minutes

Servings: 10

Ingredients:

- Peanut Butter: 1 cup
- Sugar: 1 cup
- 1 Egg

Directions:

1. Blend all of the ingredients with a hand mixer.
2. Spray trays of air fryer with canola oil. (Alternatively, parchment paper can also be used, but it will take longer to cook your cookies)
3. Set the air fryer temperature to 350 degrees and preheat it.
4. Place rounded dough balls onto air fryer trays. Press down softly with the back of a fork.
5. Place air fryer tray in your air fryer in the middle place. Cook for five minutes.

6. Use milk to serve with cookies.

Nutrition: Calories – 236 Protein – 6 g. Fat – 13 g. Carbs – 26 g.

Sweet Pear Stew

Preparation Time: 10 minutes

Cooking Time: 15 minutes

Servings: 4

Ingredients:

- 4 pears, cored and cut into wedges
- 1 tsp vanilla
- 1/4 cup apple juice
- 2 cups grapes, halved

Directions:

1. Put all of the ingredients in the inner pot of air fryer and stir well.
2. Seal pot and cook on high for 15 minutes.
3. As soon as the cooking is done, let it release pressure naturally for 10 minutes then release remaining using quick release. Remove lid.
4. Stir and serve.

Nutrition: Calories – 162 Protein – 1.1 g. Fat – 0.5 g. Carbs – 41.6 g.

Vanilla Apple Compote

Preparation Time: 10 minutes

Cooking Time: 15 minutes

Servings: 6

Ingredients:

- 3 cups apples, cored and cubed
- 1 tsp vanilla
- 3/4 cup coconut sugar
- 1 cup of water
- 2 tbsp fresh lime juice

Directions:

1. Put all of the ingredients in the inner pot of air fryer and stir well.
2. Seal pot and cook on high for 15 minutes.
3. As soon as the cooking is done, let it release pressure naturally for 10 minutes then release remaining using quick release. Remove lid.
4. Stir and serve.

Nutrition: Calories – 76 Protein – 0.5 g. Fat – 0.2 g. Carbs – 19.1 g.

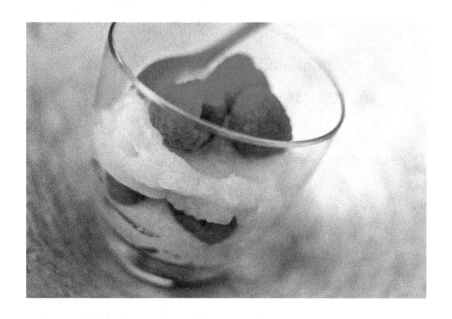

Apple Dates Mix

Preparation Time: 10 minutes

Cooking Time: 15 minutes

Servings: 4

Ingredients:

- 4 apples, cored and cut into chunks
- 1 tsp vanilla
- 1 tsp cinnamon
- 1/2 cup dates, pitted
- 1 1/2 cups apple juice

Directions:

1. Put all of the ingredients in the inner pot of air fryer and stir well.
2. Seal and cook on high for 15 minutes.
3. As soon as the cooking is done, let it release pressure naturally for 10 minutes then release remaining using quick release. Remove lid.
4. Stir and serve.

Nutrition: Calories – 226 Protein – 1.3 g. Fat – 0.6 g. Carbs – 58.6 g.

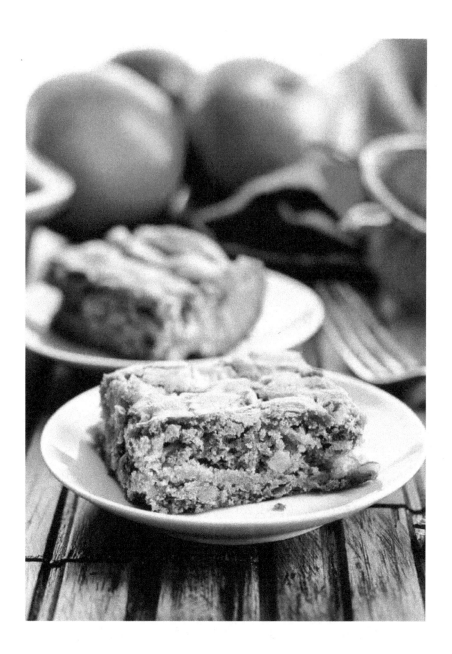

Chocolate Rice

Preparation Time: 10 minutes

Cooking Time: 20 minutes

Servings: 4

Ingredients:

- 1 cup of rice
- 1 tbsp cocoa powder
- 2 tbsp maple syrup
- 2 cups almond milk

Directions:

1. Put all of the ingredients in the inner pot of air fryer and stir well.
2. Seal pot and cook on high for 20 minutes.
3. As soon as the cooking is done, let it release pressure naturally for 10 minutes then release remaining using quick release. Remove lid.
4. Stir and serve.

Nutrition: Calories – 474 Protein – 6.3 g. Fat – 29.1 g. Carbs – 51.1 g.

Raisins Cinnamon Peaches

Preparation Time: 10 minutes

Cooking Time: 15 minutes

Servings: 4

Ingredients:

- 4 peaches, cored and cut into chunks
- 1 tsp vanilla
- 1 tsp cinnamon
- 1/2 cup raisins
- 1 cup of water

Directions:

1. Put all of the ingredients in the inner pot of air fryer and stir well.
2. Seal pot and cook on high for 15 minutes.
3. As soon as the cooking is done, let it release pressure naturally for 10 minutes then release remaining using quick release. Remove lid.
4. Stir and serve.

Nutrition: Calories – 118 Protein – 2 g. Fat – 0.5 g. Carbs – 29 g.

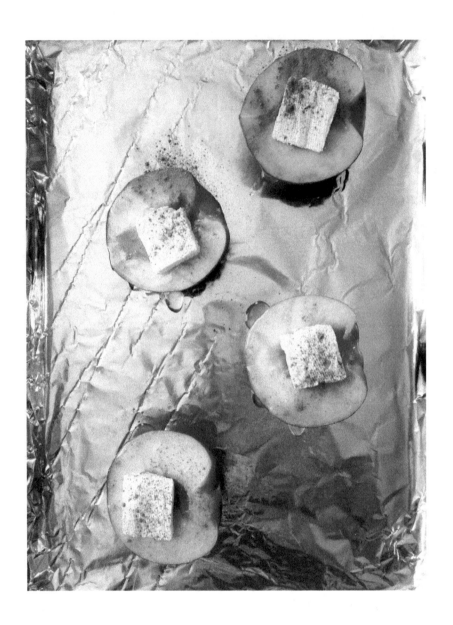

Lemon Pear Compote

Preparation Time: 10 minutes

Cooking Time: 15 minutes

Servings: 6

Ingredients:

- 3 cups pears, cored and cut into chunks
- 1 tsp vanilla
- 1 tsp liquid stevia
- 1 tbsp lemon zest, grated
- 2 tbsp lemon juice

Directions:

1. Put all of the ingredients in the inner pot of air fryer and stir well.
2. Seal pot and cook on high for 15 minutes.
3. As soon as the cooking is done, let it release pressure naturally for 10 minutes then release remaining using quick release. Remove lid.
4. Stir and serve.

Nutrition: Calories – 50 Protein – 0.4 g. Fat – 0.2 g. Carbs – 12.7

CONCLUSION

Air fryers are a relatively new piece of kitchen gadgetry. They are used by individuals who want to cook healthy foods using less oil and less fat then their conventional counterparts.

In addition to being a healthier alternative to deep frying, air fryers are also fun to use. Air-frying not only produces lots of fun and tasty food, it also saves you time and money. You can cook without the need of a griddle or a stovetop, which frees up your kitchen so you can focus on eating more healthy foods!

It is important to have an air fryer that is up to par. If you want an air fryer that will last for years, make sure that you buy an durable one. To help you choose the right air fryer for you, we have compiled a list of the best air fried ovens!

The Airfryer has several seating options. The four different versions include:

Small Seating–The size of the seating area is 13.5" x 8.5" x 9.5".

Medium Seating–The size of the seating area is 20" x 12".

Large Seating–The size of the seating area is 23" x 15".

Extra Large Seating–The size is 32" X 21". The extra large seat could accommodate up to 8 pieces. A small, medium or large fryer is included with every air fryer and can be purchased separately. The only part that may need to be purchased separately is a colander for the basket which will hold up to 16 cups depending on the size of the basket that you are using. There are no other accessories required for the air fryer: please see the specifications on this page for further details.

What's happening to our restaurant food? The answer is rather simple. We are over-cooking and over-frying foods, and most of it is for the wrong reasons.

Nobody wants to eat overcooked, undercooked, or under-salted food. Restaurant owners are turning away good customers in the name of profit.

That's not our fault. It's up to the professional chefs to do a better job with their cooking skills.

We use our Air Fryers to cook foods that don't require cooking at all. We use them to cook and heat our foods in such a way that they're ready to eat right out of the air fryer. There's no need for you to heat up your kitchen with a conventional oven or stove, just put the food in and let it finish fully. You'll be amazed at how delicious your foods can taste when you use an Air Fryer!

Today's busy lifestyle often leaves us with little time to cook. For those of you who don't have time to cook, but still need your food, the air fryer is for you.

An air fryer is an appliance that cooks food by circulating hot air over it. The circulating air causes the food to slowly cook within a sealed container while removing excess oil and fat from the food. By sealing the food in a hermetic chamber during cooking, no additional oil is released into the air. This is important because it prevents the flavor of the food from being compromised. The result is a fast and easy way to prepare delicious meals without having to use any grease or oils while eroding your pantry of oils.

In this air fryer cookbook, we will teach you how to use your air fryer most effectively and how to avoid common mistakes. From learning how to clean and maintain your air fryer to finding creative recipes, this guide will help you get the most out of your air fryer today